FITNESS THE RIGHT WAY

Your Personal Training Manual

Carlin Ashan Wilson

ISBN: 979-8-218-07102-8

Printed in the United States of America

TABLE OF CONTENTS

PREFACE

There are so many books, manuals, and articles designed to give direction to someone looking to improve their overall fitness and/or health. So, I would like to give you more insight on the steps needed to design your exercise program and more importantly, attempt to put the puzzle pieces together on what it really takes to lose weight while answering questions often left unanswered in those books, manuals, and articles.

For every piece of literature written, there is an attempt to answer the age-old question…. *How can I lose weight?* I have been a fitness trainer for over 20 years, and I have had this question presented to me by every client I have worked with. And after every consultation, *(this is where I gather information for more insight on the individual)*, I found myself giving a different answer to each client. I believe the answer peels back too many layers to only provide one simple answer(s). First, physiological contraindications may be present. The individual can be unaware of conditions such as having an underactive thyroid (*disruption of metabolic processes that leads to weight gain*) or having a food sensitivity that causes constant internal inflammation. There are many reasons a person can find it difficult to lose weight, yet we as fitness professionals attempt to simplify this question with a quick answer, which frankly, I find impossible. Even more, there are additional internal and external factors to consider such as genetics (*predisposition of cardiovascular and/or heart diseases*), current fitness levels, hectic work schedule *(hindering consistency),* dietary habits, and limited availability…. just to name a few. We all have familiarity with some, if not all these factors. It is safe to say that no programming should be prescribed prior to probing key factors like eating habits (*food sensitivities or lack of efficient digestion*), physical and/or mental barriers such as failures with past fitness programs, or mental exhaustion from attempted diets and/or weight loss programs that just would not get the job done. Without addressing these variables, even the most seasoned fitness professional would be guessing at best. Besides, the real question every weight loss seeker is asking is, "How can I lose weight as fast as possible, by either a quick fix diet or exercise routine that cuts body fat, while increasing strength so I can have the "toned" look?" This question is literally asking the fitness professional to somehow grow magic beans from the same beanstalk that has only harvested regular green beans in the past.

The function of our physiological system is much too complex to adapt that quickly to one simple remedy. Correction…. *"adapts safely and in a way that allows your body to maintain the change without some gimmick of continuing to consume supplements, a pill or a food plan that is so restrictive you couldn't possibly maintain longevity."* This is because the body is always seeking to maintain a stable internal environment, as it deals with external changes *(Homeostasis)*. As we exercise *(which is an external change),* our body's ATP cycle must generate enough fuel from our glucose/glycogen stores *(sugars/carbohydrates)* to match the energy output needed to fulfill the requirements of performing the exercise *(which is the internal change)*. This internal adaptation alone (increase in muscle tissue), forces a change in the environment thus speeding up the metabolism which promotes weight and/or body fat loss. What you have just read, is the most effective and natural way to positively reinforce weight changes that you are able to maintain throughout your life. It is this concept that I hope to elaborate in more detail throughout this manual. Throughout this read, I also hope to detail the steps needed to keep your body consistently responding to your exercise program and ensure effective results.

Unfortunately, the industry has become financially motivated and instead of giving the consumer the recipe for sustainable success, we often promote quick weight loss solutions to appease this "quick, fast and in a hurry" society, accustomed to receiving any and everything at the snap of a finger. It is a grave mistake to gratify these expectations and "we" the fitness industry must do a better job providing valuable information and tactics that promotes a lasting physical and mental health lifestyle that will undoubtedly improve the wellbeing of our clients (*consumer base*). There are yet quite a few fitness professionals promoting the proper way to implement a healthy lifestyle and we need to promote and support those individuals and/or companies.

Over the length of my career, I have maintained a very science-based approach to exercise testing and prescription and all my clients can speak to obtaining not only sustainable results but a level of understanding that empowers them to maintain even without a trainer. I develop and prescribe injury prevention - strength training programs that promote healthy joint and tissue function as well as aerobic conditioning *(using their own tailored heart rate zones to dictate energy output)*. And even when client(s) wavered or took an absence from training, they were able to hold on to my teaching methods and continue pursuing their goals. To quote some of my clients, *"It is very comforting to know that even if my schedule does not allow me to train with Carlin, I am yet able to initiate the previous plan he has given me and stay on track. This makes me feel like I have learned something over the years."* I am immensely proud of this. Mostly, to know that I have been giving them valuable information and programming that will not be an endangerment to their health and function.

Allow me to introduce myself. My name is Carlin Wilson. I have been a Fitness/Health Coach for 21 years but in addition, I obtained a Bachelor of Science in Exercise Science *(the study of the movement and the accompanying functional responses and adaptations)*, while studying within the Physical Therapy, Athletic Training and Stretch Recovery programs at Western Michigan University. I am also professor within the Movement Science program Schoolcraft College (in Livonia Michigan) and within the Wellness Health & Exercise Science program Macomb Community College in Warren Michigan. While this is unique, the exposure to multiple disciplines and programs worked out to my advantage as I evolved as a Fitness Professional. I was able to speak to consumer issues in a way that established credibility in my abilities, and afforded me the opportunity to collaborate with patients/clients no matter where they were within their journey *(post-surgery, post rehab, after injury, etc.)*

When I started in commercial fitness as a personal trainer in 2001, the industry was still riding the "group exercise" boom that started in the mid-late 80's. Consumers were enjoying cardiovascular and strength training classes that were inspiring and full of excitement. Motivated people pushing themselves to the limits of their physical capabilities together in unison and to the beat *(musical cadence)*, is very energizing. While this format was very influential in jump-starting the consumer's path to a healthy lifestyle, over the years I noticed an increase in minor/major joint and muscle ailments/injuries and an absence of proper stretching and recovery programming.

Many of us have participated in numerous exercise disciplines/plans, without knowing if the level of activity or if the type of movements were appropriate for our individual fitness level(s). This does not mean the choice of exercise discipline was wrong……It just means that you must seek to understand your own body's mechanics/contraindications and whether the movements may progressively wear and tear on joint function. The body is a highly intelligent organism and will overcompensate *(in this case,means to disproportionately utilize the left or right-side muscle(s) and/or joints causing muscular imbalances)* to protect an unsupported or weakened joint/muscle while performing a specific movement. It is not common knowledge to just understand your muscular imbalances. We are generally not made aware of any imbalances until after an injury and start engaging in some physical therapy or rehab. If you have developed muscular imbalances, you would benefit more from exercises that incorporate more sagittal planes (*exercises performed in vertical plane and divides the body into right and left side portions*) movements or unilateral training. These stabilizing exercises performed by splitting the body's left and right side will help correct imbalances and limit joint injuries and/or ailments. Therefore, a base knowledge of your muscle(s) abilities and limitations not only helps you make better decisions on which exercise classes or disciplines are a better fit but will also encourage you to implement injury prevention practices within your fitness programming.

My hope is that by the completion of this read, you will feel more confident in your understanding of basic functional exercises and corrective movements and the role they play in injury prevention. I also attempt to inform you on why the implementation of proper techniques and awareness of our bodies are necessary to ensure sustainable results, while minimizing the onset of preventable setbacks.

CHAPTER 1
HOME IS WHERE IT ALL BEGINS

Starting my path to weight loss

I am going to begin this chapter by explaining what I mean when I say, "Home is where it all begins." Instinctively most will suggest that I am referring to the place where I reside. My living quarters or my place of peace….and you would be correct. HOME (should be) is the place where you fuel your body *(eat),* rest your brain *(sleep),* and revive *(stress relievers)* yourself to prepare to manage the tasks and stresses of the outside world. That means if you are not obtaining these essential elements at HOME first, how do you expect your body to cooperate, adapt and change? Let us work our way up the list by addressing stress first.

I believe STRESS is the biggest culprit for weight gain in the world today. We all encounter stress daily. For some of us, stress constantly changes our daily plans and forces us into this repetitive cycle of mental anxiety for which our bodies internally respond with a series of hormones released into our system that (if it occurs too often within the day), can cause an increase of fat storage. In scientific language: Cortisol is a steroid hormone that helps the body respond to stress. When we are stressed (by any external or internal stimulus) Cortisol is produced and then released into our bloodstream. Our elevated level of stress triggers Cortisol to then target cells to convert stored fat, protein and carbohydrate molecules into glucose or ready energy. It is then that we enter "Fight or Flight" mode (*a term I am sure most of you have heard before)*. The setback with having repeated stress episodes of Fight or Flight mode is that any unused energy is automatically stored back into our system as fat. This is the reason we tend to gain weight *(Increased body fat content)* when we are constantly stressed. Not to mention Cortisol increases our blood sugar levels and controls our sleep/wake cycle. We all know how important sleep and managing our blood sugar level impacts our weight management. Below, I have listed a few activities to help reduce the effects of the daily stressors:

Stress Relief Activities

1. **Compartmentalize what a real stress threat is** (freeway traffic to work is a daily occurrence and should not affect because there isn't anything you can do about it. You cannot quit your job because of traffic and unsafe drivers. Find a tactic to deal with daily occurrences such as soft music or audiobooks to stimulate meditation and calmness).

2. **Leave work at work** (do not bring work negativity to your home conversation or thoughts)

3. **Spend/devote attention to family** (participate in family fitness activities together as well as relaxation time)

4. **Find a quiet space to yourself** (30 minutes of mental health meditation)

Sleep Improvement - Getting 7 hours of sleep will:

1. **Get 7 hours of sleep per night**

a. Reduces stress and improve mood

b. Boost immune system, (*drink jasmine, or ginger tea 30 minutes before bedtime)*

c. Will prevent weight gain

   i. When your body does not get enough rest, the body produces Ghrelin (*which is a hormone that boosts our appetites*). Can you relate to eating late just because you cannot sleep? I can…

b. Improves Concentration during your workouts

   i. Sleep improves higher cognitive function, increasing reaction time and muscle recovery. Contrary to this fact, sleep deprivation negatively impacts strength and power

Nutrition Habits

1. **Eat 5-6 small, portioned meals per day** (eat something nutritious every 3 to 3.5 hours assuming you are awake 16 hours per day)

2. **Make sure to investigate and find out the foods you are sensitive to** (food sensitivity blood work with your doctor)

3. **Make sure to drink at least 115 – 120 ounces per day**

These three components are necessary to stimulate sustainable weight loss and/or fitness conditioning. We need the discipline to maintain them. Easier said than done right? I know, but we must remember that the human body works as a unit. If we do not implement selfcare tactics, the body's response to any attempt to exercise will be less than favorable. Fact is, the body's response to exercise is only favorable when we get ample sleep, eat nutritious foods, and perform mental stress relief activities daily.

In the preface, we talked about addressing barriers that can prevent adopting consistent exercise and proper eating habits. Now is the time to really sit down and examine what they are, if any. Below, is a list of barriers to consider before moving on to program implementation:

- **Time** (what time of the day can you carve out 1 hour for exercise and 30 minutes for mental and physical recovery?)

    - Before work? After work? Middle of the day?

- **Hectic schedule** (any support system for your children or other mandatory tasks?)

    - Working multiple jobs?
    - Daily tasks full, no previous need or desire to carve out any "me time"

- Previous Injuries or ailments

    - Any difficulties completing physical daily tasks?

- Have you been advised medically to avoid certain movements?
- Previous orthopedic injuries or surgeries? Did you receive physical therapy?

- **Mental Readiness** (what is your motivation?)

  - Seeking superficial change only?
  - Medically advised to lose weight.
  - Have you internally accepted the discipline it will take to succeed?

Once you have answered and addressed these questions, you are ready to begin prescribing yourself, your workout plan. The Guideline to planning a personal exercise program consist of addressing 4 components:

- **Regularity:** Which is establishing the number of times per week you intent to exercise

  - 4-5 days per week (is required for weight loss)

- **Effort % :** Answers how "hard" to exercise

  - 60%-70% intensity is desirable for weight loss (explained more in heart rate zones calculation in chapter 3)

- **Time Period:** Amount of time per exercise session

  - 60 minutes recommended for weight loss

- **Exercise Category:** Which exercise discipline is performed?

  - Bodyweight/Functional Training program is recommended by me and will explain more in chapter 2

The *Regularity* or number of days you should workout is very subjective to the individual and its effectiveness depends on the individual's consistency along with stretching and muscle recovery sessions. During my bodybuilding years, I trained 4 days per week with 2 additional days consisting of mobility, stretching and recovery activities. So, in total, I trained/recovered 6 days per week. YES, stretching and mobility exercises count as training days. Giving your muscles the opportunity to recover and heal is an especially important component of training ….in any capacity whether that's basketball, gymnastics, bodybuilding etc,..

If you are a beginner just starting your journey, I would recommend 3 days of resistance and cardiovascular training along with 2 days of stretching and muscle recovery activities. Leaving two days free of any activities to allow muscles to acclimate to the additional stress placed on the muscle tissue and for you to get through what is likely to be at least 3 weeks of muscle soreness and/or possible muscle spasms.

Effort % refers to an estimated training intensity percentage relative to your maximal strength. An example would be explained as follows:

- You are able to complete 15 pushups before total failure (the 16th pushup you were not able to push all the up).

- You want to train at the **65%** intensity recommended

- You then set out to figure the total # of pushups you need to complete in order to fulfill 65% of your 1 set max (**15 pushups x .65**) = 9.75 or **10 total pushups.**

- Now your prescription is 3-4 sets of 10 repetitions (pushups)

"<u>Period</u>" is set at a minimum of 60 min. For weight loss, I recommend splitting the time so 30 minutes is dedicated to cardiovascular activities and 30 minutes reserved for resistance training activities. The *"<u>Exercise Category</u>"* is easily described as the activity discipline you choose. Whether that's CrossFit, Weight Training, Circuit Training, or Interval Training……they all are explained under each training principle.

It is particularly important to understand that when you intend to make any meaningful changes in your life, you must alter your environment (especially at home) in order to ensure success. Changing your environment requires tough decisions and may require you to adjust home habits that affect your children and/or spouse. You may have to make schedule adjustments to accommodate your exercise time(s). When you find a workout time that suits you, you must stick with it and hopefully you are able to maneuver your daily tasks and appointments around that time.

I am often asked, what time of day is the best time to work out? I personally encourage the early morning workout. You can jump start your day and supply yourself with enough energy to get through your hectic day. Now you will have to monitor your bedtime and make sure it is early enough for you to get those 7 hours of sleep required in order to make an early morning session work. This is a tough adjustment for the first 2 weeks or so, but your body will adjust to the new wakeup schedule and your body will look forward to your early morning workouts. Now on the contrary, a midday or evening workout can be very much effective, however you must be aware of the late afternoon meal, coupled with the afternoon crash that can have you feeling sluggish. You are likely to skip an evening workout and go home after a long workday and a heavy meal on your stomach. If you choose to start with an evening workout schedule, be flexible and open to trying the morning, if an evening schedule does not work. Remember, the important thing is that you fit your workout in your day.

Earlier in this chapter, I presented a couple of nutrition habits that are important to implement when starting a consistent exercise program. One of them was to eat 5-6 small, portioned meals throughout your day. Now, it is my experience that daily moderate-intensity exercising will help stimulate your metabolism to speed up, thus requiring an increase in appetite. Unless you have access to a licensed dietitian or nutrition specialist who can fully guide you on any major changes to your eating habits, I recommend one simple task …..and that's to clean out the refrigerator. Rid your refrigerator and kitchen pantry of all white flour products, sugars products (*aspartame, dextrose, high fructose corn*), and any processed foods (*food that is premade then either dumped into sodium water or hydrogenated oils to be preserved*). You replace those food items with Lean Meats, Fruits, Vegetables, and Whole

Foods/Grains (*food grown in a garden*). This may take some creativity if you have children in the home, but you must find a way to maintain these adjustments so that you are feeding your body nutritious foods that will support your newly implemented, daily exercise routine.

CHAPTER 2
START WITH THE BASICS

6 basic movements of Bodyweight Training

Basic Bodyweight Training is a very understated type/style of Resistance Training. I believe that the absence of proper bodyweight training principles could very well be a likely reason joint and muscle injuries are more and more prevalent. We all perform 6 basic body movements (squat, lunge, lift, pull, push and press) daily, yet we often neglect these basic moves within our workout routine. Between adding weights such as kettlebells and medicine balls, and implementing more weighted compound movements, I believe the various complexities of these movements have changed in a way that the consumer loses track of the basic mechanics of each basic movement. Nothing against compound exercises and I believe they are beneficial and part of functional training. I'm just imploring that we continue to remind the consumer of proper mechanics in our teachings. I ask myself the question.... " *if we place more emphasis on the mechanics of basic movements within our workout routines, would we experience less joint and muscle injuries?* "

Advancements in the fitness industry stimulate growth in our attempt to aid the consumer in taking the necessary steps to increase quality of life as we age. However, we must not neglect the importance of consistently performing the 6 basic movements within our exercise routines to decrease the likelihood of injury. The body is a kinetic chain of muscle, bones and tissues interacting with joints to perform movements. *(5 kinetic chain checkpoints) are: 1. feet/ankles, 2. knees, 3. hip/pelvis, 4. shoulders, 5. head)* Meaning, if your hamstrings are tight (restrictive hip extension), then there will be complications with hip flexion (bending over) movements, not to mention the stress you are putting on your lower back and lumbar region (*spinal cord*). Which inversely means, if you do not practice hamstring lengthening exercises such as the airplane stretch (*mimics bending over, picking up an object) or* stiff legged deadlift, you can be subject to tightening of the lower pelvic/hip function or worse, experience sciatic nerve issues. The fact is, if we do not implement these exercises/stretches on our own, we will more than likely be forced to eventually perform them for the physical therapist *(after experiencing an injury)*. If you are receiving physical therapy, then you have already suffered an injury and/or endured surgery to a joint or muscle. We often blame joint and/or muscle tears or injuries on fluke accidents. Contrary to that thought, fluke accidents involving muscle or joint injuries are rare and most injuries are more likely the source of neglect and/or overuse.

Bodyweight training itself, involves any exercise or movement performed using your own bodyweight and gravity as resistance. When I look at this closely, I come to the realization that this is pretty much everyday life. From the simplest act of walking outside in a brisk wind all the way to kneeling over your bathtub to clean, the usage of our muscles for daily life activities are a necessity. However, for some reason we tend to gravitate to exercise disciplines where resistance weight is added (ex. Dumbbell, Kettlebell, Barbell weight just to name a few) BEFORE perfecting Bodyweight (or Functional) Training. Now let's discuss neglect and overuse of muscles and joint function.

Neglect sounds intentional, but in most cases, it just means *oversight*. Lack of knowledge and information or just the incomplete gathering of information can cause us to do harm to our bodies when our intentions are just to get stronger and feel better. Truth is, there are some exercise practices that must be performed to replicate daily activities with greater ease and protect ourselves from overuse injuries. You really can't just, "do what you want" in the gym. When you purchase a car, your intent may be to sustain effective operation of the car well past 200,000 miles. It really doesn't matter how clean you keep the outside of the car, if you do not keep up with the oil changes and engine/transmission maintenance, the car will eventually cease to operate regardless of your goal. The body works the same way. If your job requires you to lift boxes for 6-8 hours per day and you do not properly train and stretch your legs and abdominals by replicating squats and deadlifts, you will soon wear down your back and eventually become unable to meet the physical demands of the job. Yes! Training muscles is a form of injury prevention. You will increase muscle endurance, allowing you to perform repetitive movements for long periods of time using proper technique.

When we do not train our muscles to bear the workload of performing numerous daily tasks/positions, we are vulnerable to the onset of injuries. This is due to fatigue setting within the muscle, then forcing the joint and muscle to continue to perform the movement, which sacrifices proper mechanics. Why does a basketball player practice for hours on hours in the offseason? Most will say to improve at the mechanics of the game itself (shooting form, plyometrics, agility drills, etc.) and you would be correct but that's not the only reason. Another important reason is to condition their bodies to resist fatigue and be effective in performing those skills at a high level for 48 minutes. The fluidity of your jump shot, the balance to tip toe the out of bounds line, or just to defensively stay in front of your opponent for 48 minutes, all depends on your level of conditioning. The greatest shooter in the world will miss shots late in the game due to fatigue. If your legs feel heavy, how can you jump? In other words, if you do not condition your muscles to handle workload without undue fatigue, your effectiveness will be marginal. You may be asking, *"what does it mean to condition?"* Webster dictionary explains conditioning as the "state of physical fitness or readiness for use." You are preparing your body for workload and/or resistance it may endure. Athletes perform/practice specific training protocols to maximize the use of the primary muscles used during that activity. Interestingly enough, the same rule of thumb should apply to everyone…. Not just athletes.

Many of you have experienced ailments such as chronic lower back pain, strains, sprains, tendonitis, just to name a few. Before you just give in to the notion that the cause of this pain is from getting older….well think about your job. Do you have a manual labor job that causes you to perform the same or similar repetitive movements for long periods of time? If this doesn't describe you, then think of a physical hobby or chore that has your body in a position for long periods of time and is difficult to sustain. Are you thinking? Now let me ask you this question… Do you believe your lower back was created strong enough to hold your bodyweight upright all day *without* daily strengthening your core muscles (Abdominals, Pelvic, Lower back, and Hip muscles) through exercise? I will let you in on something I realized about a year into my profession: our muscles perform the lifting duties while our joints allow the up, down, and side to side movements. Basically, we should not be lifting, pushing, or pulling with our joints. Joints are not muscles and should not be used as such. Daily practices of bodyweight movements and exercises stimulate a consistent flow of blood throughout all extremities (legs and arms), transporting oxygen. Oxygen improves the function of joints (cartilage, ligaments, and tendons) and promotes healthy muscle tissue. It is this specific occurrence that minimizes the onset of chronic muscles and joint discomfort.

10 Reasons Body Weight Training is effective

- **Increases Muscles and Joints Strength**

  - Significantly reduces stress on hips, knees, and ankles

- **Improves Posture**

  - Better circulation
  - Promotes spine and neck health

- **Enhances Balance and Mobility**

  - Reduced risk of injury

- **Boosts Endurance and Increase Performance**

  - Decreased risk of cardiovascular disease

- **Burns More Calories**

  - Promotes Weight Loss

- **Support Muscle Growth**

- Speeds up metabolism

- **Improves Flexibility**

  - Less Pain
  - Increased range of motion

- **Builds a Strong Core**

  - Enhances Balance and Stability

- **Doesn't require much space and pieces of equipment**

  - Low Cost

- **Adaptable and enjoyable**

  - Versatile style of Training

Are these reasons enough to stimulate an interest in focusing more on Basic Movement Training? I sure hope so. I have attached a link to this book (QR Code located on the back page) that contains a 30 min video describing the details of all 6 basic movements as well grant you access to all paid content and videos on my website. Please follow and implement into your full body workout routine to achieve measurable results.

CHAPTER 3
"CARDIO" INTO YOUR PROPER HEART RATE ZONE

(Let your Heart Rate dictate how you Train)

This is a very interesting topic because I believe that the exercise enthusiast is aware of this notion that working out within a tailored heart rate training zone is beneficial to conditioning (adaptation) and to maximize fat loss however, for some reason it's just not practiced. The most interesting thing I have noticed is that with the exception of the athlete, most of us track our heart rate just to make sure we don't die (metaphorically) during the workout Lol! (heart rate exceeding 185 bpm or above). Think about the last fitness class or activity you participated in that left you feeling depleted of energy and not able to sustain the pace as long as you wanted to. Now, do you recall seeing another participant complete the activity/class without being as winded or out of breath? It appears they coasted through the workout. The difference between you and that person is conditioning. The other participant has spent more time training at an elevated heart rate therefore their body has adapted, now promoting optimal caloric expenditure. This is where we all desire to be, however, the proper steps must be taken.

First, you must invest in a heart rate tracking device. There are so many inexpensive options you pretty much can just take your pick. The tracker only needs to be able to calculate calories burned, heart rate and track steps. The step tracker really motivates to keep you moving, reducing your shut-down time, and stimulating improved blood circulation throughout the day. We all are aware of the advantages of tracking calories burned. Just the caloric expenditure daily goal alone is enough to keep us scheduling workouts. The question is "HOW" do we meet our caloric expenditure goals in the most effective way? I mean anyone can just start running until they can't go anymore but are those calories burned efficiently? Is that the blueprint for hitting your goal? In almost every case that answer is NO. The fact is, we all have an optimal heart rate training zone that allows us to burn predominantly fat calories. I am going to help each of you find that training zone by using the equation below:

1. First, take your resting heart rate, using your carotid artery (neck) or ulna (wrist) for three (3) consecutive mornings in a row because every morning may be different, and this will enable you to get a more accurate average. It is very important to take your resting heart rate first thing in the morning before you get out of bed and start moving. Once you find your pulse, hold for 60 seconds (1 full minute) and record the beats.

   a. Resting heart rate on first morning:
      _________________________ beats/minute

   b. Resting heart rate on second morning:
      _________________________ beats/ minute

   c. Resting heart rate on third morning:
      _________________________beats/minute

2. Then find the average of those 3 trials (adding all the 3 trials and dividing by 3), You now have your Average Resting Heart Rate (RHR in beats per minute)

3. Now find your Heart Rate Reserve (which is your Maximum Heart Rate minus your Resting Heart Rate)

   a. 220 – your age = Maximum Heart Rate
   b. Maximum Heart Rate – Resting Heart Rate (RHR) = Heart Rate Reserve

4. Next you must determine the percentage of your max heart rate you aspire to workout in. (From my numerous teachings and certifications, I have learned that it is recommended that the novice (beginner) fitness devotee trains between *60 -70 % of their Max Heart Rate)*

5. Heart Rate Reserve multiplied (x) by .60 (60%) + Resting Heart Rate (RHR) = Lower Heart Rate Zone

6. Heart Rate Reserve multiplied (x) by .70 (70%) + Resting Heart Rate (RHR) = Upper Heart Rate Zone

(Sample Equation)

I have a Resting Heart Rate 3-day average of 61
220 – (age of 42) = 178 MHR
178(MHR) - 61(RHR) = 117 bpm (HRR)
117 (HRR) x .60 + 61 = 131bpm (Lower Zone)
117 (HRR) x .70 + 61= 143 bpm (Upper Zone)

My optimal training zone is between 131 – 143 beats per minute. It would benefit me to adjust all exercise activities so I can stay within this zone. In this zone my body doesn't have to work as hard, so I am able to perform longer and optimize fat burning. If you are a little confused by this statement, think about an airplane for a minute. When does the airplane burn more fuel? A plane burns almost 40% more fuel on takeoff than at altitude. The plane uses its engines at full power to climb to altitude but at altitude (cruise control), the plane travels easier as the air thins, thus burning less fuel. Our bodies during exercise kind of work the same way.

If we stay at a higher heart rate during exercise, we burn through our sugars (carbohydrates) quickly (term referred to as "hitting the wall"), resulting in depletion and the need to burn an alternate source of energy. It is at this point that most consumers believe the body will burn fat as an energy source at this higher heart rate, but this is not entirely true. The most readily source of energy when we have depleted our sugars is proteins. We as humans operate in a state of Catabolism (which is the process of molecules being broken down in the body to use for energy). There are 4 stages of Catabolism and the final stage is fat breakdown of adipose tissue. However, before we get to the state, we will use glycogen and proteins within the first 3 stages. This means proteins are the next most readily source of energy after sugars when the body is exerting at a higher heart rate (like the airplane take off) NOT fat. To optimize fat, you must operate longer at a sustainable (heart rate at which you can maintain consistency) heart rate. When the body is working but not too hard, your energy source will more likely be fat. So, cater your exercises so you can stay in your heart rate zone, sustain a more consistent flow of blood through the body, take less breaks (which causes the heart rate to drop too low) and operate at cruise control so your body can adjust its fuel source to your liking. Now let's talk about the primary fitness discipline that should be performed if you are looking to improve your conditioning and maximize your muscle adaptation to decrease your body fat. Cardiorespiratory Fitness is the discipline we are looking for here. I realize that there are fitness professionals and exercise disciplines that are now promoting this notion that there is no need for cardiorespiratory fitness activities, but I am NOT one of them. There is a substantial scientific study that confirms how necessary cardiovascular activities are for maximum performance as well as sustainable body fat loss. Now let's talk about the purpose of cardiorespiratory activities.

Cardiorespiratory Exercise *(aerobic exercise)* is the ability of the cardiovascular and respiratory systems to supply oxygen and nutrients to large muscle groups and sustain dynamic activity. Cardio *(refers to the distribution/transportation of oxygen)* and Respiratory *(refers to gas exchange, exhalation of Carbon Dioxide and inhalation of Oxygen)* collaborate to not only increase the overall function of the heart and lungs but increase physical conditioning. Aerobic means "with oxygen", or consistent blood volume without any disruption or stoppage *(stoppage: resulting in a drop of our heart rate)* to the flow of oxygen traveling throughout the system. In simpler terms, any sporadic or significant changes in volume (amount) of blood carrying oxygen through our system or if you break too long to catch your breath, you are now training in an Anaerobic Capacity. NOT Aerobic. Anaerobic means "without oxygen". These activities are shorter in duration and require sudden bursts of energy. Think about your previous workouts….Now based on these 2 definitions, which type of exercise(s) are you performing? If you are looking to lose weight, you will need to make the adjustment to more aerobic activities like Stairmaster, Treadmill, Elliptical, Power Walk, or Jogging. Whether the exercises are electrically powered, or manually powered, it is the continuance of moving that constitutes aerobic activity. Protocols for these devices are solely based on what you are comfortable with. First, just focus on getting your system adjusted to the length of time by starting with 20-minute sessions working your way up to

60 min sessions. Remember to let your heart rate determine how fast or slow you move. The goal is to stay within your (previously calculated) target heart rate zone, while sustaining your blood flow with aerobic activities. In addition to efficient weight loss, more important benefits of cardiorespiratory endurance activities include:

- Increases oxygen delivery to muscles

- Improves the transfer and use of oxygen

- Improves the body's ability to use energy efficiently

- Reduced risk of heart diseases

- Reduced risk of type 2 diabetes

CHAPTER 4
CONSISTENCY IS A 4-LETTER WORD
(HARD)

Consistency is a concept I believe we all grasp but find it very difficult to maintain. Even though we experience the ebbs and flows of stability within quite a few areas of our life, I believe we find it most difficult to be consistent with maintaining a daily exercise/activity routine. Why is this true? What really gets in the way of us sustaining consistency?

It would be very easy to blame the COVID-19 pandemic as the reason why most of us found it difficult to maintain a steady exercise routine. In 2018 (Pre-Pandemic), approximately 61 million Americans had gym memberships. At the time, that reflected only 19% of the total population. Which means 81% of the population either found a way to stay active at home (outdoors) or didn't exercise at all. My point for stating this is that even with the temporary closing of the gyms, only 19% of the population had to adjust to a drastic change in the process of which they exercised. So even if 50% out of the total population (very generous estimate) didn't exercise at all, 31% yet found a way to stay active without a gym membership. So, is it true that maintaining a consistent exercise routine is difficult? Let's address some factors that we must consider.

Thinking back on client experiences, I recall some explanations given that made exercising daily difficult. Work, not enough time in the day, or difficulty starting a diet. Does any of this sound familiar? Can you relate to one or more?

I have a 2-word solution to those of you who feel like the previous setbacks given speaks to how you feel…. SELF CARE. Self-Care through physical and mental relief activities are important and under-practiced by society, especially for Generation X (born between 1965-1980), Baby Boomers (born between 1946-1964) and a large portion of the Millennials (born between 1981 – 1996). I have consulted many clients and I almost always have gotten "NO" answers to these questions,

1. Do you treat yourself to a massage at least once per month?

2. Do you take time off outside of holiday paid time off?

3. Do you get outside and walk or just get some sun at least 30 min per day?

My next question is: "So, let me get this straight, you don't get any fresh air on a daily basis, you don't take physical and/or mental health breaks from work and you have never had a massage to release tension from your body and now you want to use that formula to help you lose weight and get physically fit?" Some of you reading this book have minimal knowledge of fitness and what it takes to develop a fitness regimen and even you know this expectation doesn't sound right. You absolutely cannot lose weight with that lifestyle practice.

Earlier in chapter 1, we addressed stress, sleep and nutrition as very important components that must be attended to before the body can make the proper adaptations needed to change your body composition (lose weight). It is very difficult to find consistency in any area of our lives if we are stressed out. Stress causes overeating, lack of quality sleep and irritability that continues to throw our hormones in a tailspin and unable to find stability. Let's reduce some of the frustration that comes with trying to stay consistent. First answer these questions for yourself:

- **What equipment do you have access to?**

  - Home exercise equipment and space makes it easier to get your workouts in without the pressure to schedule gym visits.

- **What exercise discipline interests you?**

  - Find a discipline that interests you but remember to account for your own muscle/joint contraindications (concerns) and staying within your calculated heart rate zones

- **Will you let barriers hold you back?**

  - Are you mentally ready to push through variables outside of your control and commit to exercising daily no matter what?

- **Is accountability your strong suit?**

  - Can you achieve this with no one looking at you or after you? Don't be afraid to ask for assistance.

Once you have the answers to these questions, then consider these tips before starting your fitness programming:

1. Starting an exercise program is an important decision. But it doesn't have to be an overwhelming one. By planning carefully and pacing yourself, you can establish a healthy habit that lasts a lifetime.

2. Consider your fitness goals. Are you starting a fitness program to help lose weight? Or do you have another motivation, such as preparing for a marathon? Having clear goals can help you gauge your progress and stay motivated.

3. Understanding the body's adaptation *(soreness and/or lactic acid buildup in the muscle tissue)* to exercise and placing an emphasis on recovery is vital to your ability to stay motivated and reach your goal.

4. You might consider using fitness apps for smart devices or other activity tracking devices, such as ones that can track your distance, track calories burned or monitor your heart rate.

5. Start slowly and build up gradually. Give yourself plenty of time to warm up and cool down with easy walking or gentle stretching. Then speed up to a pace you can continue for five to 10 minutes without getting overly tired. As your stamina improves, gradually increase the amount of time you exercise. Work your way up to 30 to 60 minutes of exercise most days of the week.

6. Start low and progress slowly. If you're just beginning to exercise, start cautiously and progress slowly. Listen to your body. If you feel pain, shortness of breath, dizziness or nausea, take a break. You may be pushing yourself too hard.

7. Be flexible. If you're not feeling good, give yourself permission to take a day or two off.

8. Break things up if you have to. You don't have to do all your exercise at one time, so you can weave in activity throughout your day. Shorter but more-frequent sessions have aerobic benefits, too. Exercising in short sessions a few times a day may fit into your schedule better than a single 30-minute session. Any amount of activity is better than none at all.

9. If you have an injury or a medical condition, consult your doctor or an exercise therapist for help designing a fitness program that gradually improves your range of motion, strength, and endurance.

10. Allow time for recovery. Many people start exercising with frenzied zeal — working out too long or too intensely — and give up when their muscles and joints become sore or injured. Plan time between sessions for your body to rest and recover.

11. Build activity into your daily routine. Finding time to exercise can be a challenge. To make it easier, schedule time to exercise as you would any other appointment.

12. Plan to alternate among activities that emphasize different parts of your body, such as walking, swimming and strength training.

13. If listening to music doesn't suit you, plan to watch your favorite show while walking on the treadmill, read while riding a stationary bike, or take a break to go on a walk at work.

14. If you lose motivation, set new goals or try a new activity. Exercising with a friend or taking a class at a fitness center may help, too.

15. If you're planning to invest in exercise equipment, choose something that's practical, enjoyable and easy to use. You may want to try out certain types of equipment at a fitness center before investing in your own equipment.

16. You'll probably start with athletic shoes. Be sure to pick shoes designed for the activity you have in mind. For example, running shoes are lighter in weight than cross-training shoes, which are more supportive.

17. Anticipate barriers and/or stumbling blocks to your change, such as overambitious goals and self-defeating beliefs and attitudes....BLOCK OUT ALL NEGATIVITY!

This book is not meant to deter you from hiring a certified fitness professional. I recommend the assistance of a fitness professional to maximize your results. A professional, degreed, and certified trainer can help you achieve benchmarks you may not be able to do alone. The expertise of a professional fitness trainer has premium value when determining the proper exercise discipline to use based on your needs and past injuries and/or muscle and joint concerns. You wouldn't hire an attorney to defend your child without that lawyer having passed the bar and obtaining a law degree, right? Why would you hire an uneducated/uncertified personal trainer? Or worse, attempt to change/develop your exercise program without proper direction?

Remember to make sure you explore all signs the body gives to indicate something is off. Never ignore warning signs meant to alert you to something is awry. All explanations I have given represent how the body should respond. If your body does not respond in its proper manner, that means you could possibly have something going on internally that requires the attention of a doctor or specialist.

Thank you for reading this book and I hope this read is helpful to your fitness/health journey. Till next time.